WINNING RESOLUTIONS
A Treatise

CHARLES MWEWA

DEDICATION

To all those who seek to be the change they
want.

CONTENTS

AUTHOR'S WORD

Every year people make resolutions. So, there is an implicit understanding that resolutions are good. Indeed, they are good. Resolutions aim to self-better, self-improve, and self-actualize. These are the three ultimate objectives of any resolution.

This brief treatise provides a very nuanced but pointed debriefing on the veracity of resolutions. It is quintessentially a subtle debrief because people attempt to make resolutions and, unfortunately, majority of them fail each year. One of the reasons why they fail is addressed in this book – the lack of understanding of what a resolution is in the first place.

The book can be read and completed in less than 30 minutes, but its saliences may be endeared for years to come. Because the reader will know and appreciate the core of resolutions and the steps required to make *winning* resolutions. Be the first witness to this.

c.m.

RESOLUTIONS

Definition

The decision, the promise to yourself to do and not to do something. Resolutions are not visions of future action, or missions to be carried out, or actionable plans, or expected endeavors; they are all of the above. They are a *resolve* to make something happen, a strategy of how something is going to be done.

Elements

There are four elements of a resolution. These are:

1. It is a promise
2. To yourself
3. To act in a certain way
4. To achieve an objective

Assumption of a Decision

In every definition of a resolution, a decision is assumed. Resolutions are premised on an assumption of decisiveness. Thus, a resolution is not a trial-and-error exercise or a supposition; it is a matter of fact. It is a genuine, strong and end-of-the-cut decision that is made or reached for something to be done. They outlive visions, dreams and plans. They are declarations of fact rather than of only intentions. Once they have been declared, a decision is made, and the next phase must entail the implementation of the decision. Resolutions prefocus decisive actions.

Implementation Drive

Because resolutions presume decisiveness and must be implemented to be efficacious, they are sustained by an implementation drive. Unlike group projects or business plans which may need an external directing or implementation force, resolutions are not contingent upon any external force. Resolutions draw upon individual energies, determination and forte to their implementation. In other words, they are individual-driven.

To be implementable, resolutions require four factors:

1. Decisiveness
2. Discipline
3. Determination
4. Dutifulness

One must be decisive, disciplined, determined and dutiful to bring a resolution to its realization. These four factors must all be present if a resolution is to happen. The absence of decisiveness brings down a resolution – because resolutions assume decision-making. Lack of discipline will either lead to non-action or will abort the resolution.

Discipline is essential not only because it is necessary to the beginning of the project, but also because it is to its end. Where there is no discipline, the promise will fall completely through negligence or abandonment. One enemy of discipline is lack of setting realistic, interesting goals.

It is important that the resolutioner finds joy in those things which, while achieving the greater *agenda*, they are also enjoying the process.

Prioritization comes to mind. If possible, the resolution must be written down and the order in which it is going to be carried out.

Other strategies might include setting alarms, entrusting it unto someone one trusts to provide oversight or reminders, etc. Since resolutions are personal missions, the end result is individualistic, even if another person provided oversight.

And if the subject is not determined, any wanton discouragement or temptation will derail or even end the process. And every resolutioner (a person who resolves to do something), must know that they have a duty to monitor and feed the process towards goal accomplishment.

For example, a person who resolves to stop a bad habit by the end of the year, must decide to end that year with a positive outcome; must be disciplined enough not to slack or give in to temptations; must be determined to put in the required effort; and must have a duty to make themselves do something to achieve what they have resolved.

Resolutions are not chance game or wishes. Chances and wishes draw upon the drive or energy of an external force; resolutions on that of an internal force. Thus, the resolutioner is the progenitor and executor of their own intent. If they fail in anyone of these factors, the project called a resolution will fail.

Decisiveness and determination are very important triggers. Sometimes, a resolution may fail because it was never initiated in the first place. Decisiveness and determination will ensure that the person actually puts their hand to the peddle. Discipline and duty are necessary to ensuring that the project is carried out to the resolute end.

Fundamentals of a Promise or ACE

ACE stands for:

1. Assurance
2. Certainty
3. Expectation

A promise stands or falls on ACE. To ACE a promise, one must be assured, certain, and expect.

First, they must have assurance. Resolutions are sureties that it is possible to be held accountable for the failure to perform. They entail possibility and necessity. It is possible to undertake a resolution because there is assurance that it shall be performed. Lack of this assurance is tantamount to a wishy-washy sentimentality. People who lack this assurance must not undertake a resolution because it will lead to frustration, a mockery of one's efforts, time and thought. In other words, a resolution is a *sure* promise to oneself.

Second, there must be certainty that the resolution is a promissory note which is as good as done. In other words, a resolution is a *certain* promise to oneself.

Third, and last, a resolution must be earnestly expected. It cannot be a doubtful endeavor, but a decisive, resolved endeavor.

The idea of earnest expectation engenders performance. The resolution must happen no matter what. When it is made, it is already taken into consideration that expected impediments and detours and discouragements will arise. But the resolutioner is readily prepared to defeat all difficulties along the way. In other words, a resolution is an *earnestly expected* promise to oneself.

The Principle of Self-Assurance

A resolution is a promise made to oneself. It can be secretive or publicly made, but it must be made by and for oneself. The beneficiary is self, not directly another. The person who makes a resolution is doing it in the interest of self and in the context of self-fulfillment, and not for another.

The question is not, "Can I do this so that another can benefit?" but rather, "Can I do this that I can benefit myself to benefit others?"

So, resolutions are duty-bound, are ethically based, and are humanely efficacious. The betterment, improvement or actualization of oneself, is the duty and meaning of a resolution. These, once realized, would make the resolutioner useful and essential to the process or to others. The *mantra* is, first improving self, then another.

The principle is akin to the falling plane conception. A parent ought to make sure that they are themselves well secured in gas masks to assist their little ones. Otherwise, both may perish. Therefore, one cannot effectively serve or help others unless they are well-equipped, assured and secured themselves.

Thus, resolutions can be made for anything – religious reasons, work performance reasons, personal growth reasons, physical fitness reasons, familial reasons, etc. Rich people must make resolutions, and so should the poor. Educated people must make resolutions, and so should the uneducated. Older people as well as young people must make resolution. In other words, everyone must *reassure* themselves to *assure* others.

The Principle of Action-Orientation

The toughest part of any resolution is not the mental processes that went into it but it is the action required to make its implementation possible. One must carry out the promise by doing certain activities for a resolution to be realized. Anyone can dream and can make bold declarations. Anyone can jot down their resolutions on paper. Anyone can announce what they intend to achieve. However, it is only those who *do*, who actually achieve their objectives.

One must *do* what they promised themselves to do. They must do so decisively, deliberately, and dutifully. They must be their own bosses, managers and disciplinarians.

To do so, they must honor their own promises and work hard and smart to carry out their objectives. When it comes to resolutions, deeds and *not* words, value more. The resolutioner must do, act and perform deeds to realize their objectives.

Objectives of a Resolution

There are three objectives of a resolution:

1. Self-betterment
2. Self-improvement
3. Self-actualization

Simply put, resolutions are made to fix a deficiency, to ameliorate a condition, or to solve an urgent or immediate problem. The end is to better, improve and actualize an individual. This done, they can be confident, reassured and motivated to be who they are and become what they want to become. Those are the essences of objective resolutions.

Objectives are based on the concept of goal setting and realization. To be achievable, goals must be realistic, measurable, manageable and time-sensitive. Resolutions must follow that trajectory.

Resolutions are defined by their objectives. Objectives can vary from individual to individual. However, all objectives must have the following four characteristics:

Sense of urgency – that is, they are treated as emergencies and a response is required immediately.

Cogent – that is, they must be clear, logical, and convincing.

Relevant – that is, they are significant and meaningful.

And a sense of permanence – that is, they are timed, fixed, measured and reviewable by duration.

Resolutions cannot be open-ended, for if so, they will lack accountability and measurability. For example, an objective must include the definition of the problem to be solved, the period of time it must be resolved, and the expected results.

Reasons for Resolutions

The reasons for resolutions are as wide as the East is from the West. The most common ones include, for:

- New year's
- Fitness
- Finances
- Mental health
- Weight loss or gain
- Dietary improvements
- Family time and bonding
- Stopping or lessening habits like drug use, smoking or alcohol consumption
- Spiritual renewal
- Acquisition of new skills
- Learning new things
- Reading more
- Traveling more
- Vacationing more
- Cooking new recipes
- Volunteering
- Home decorating
- Decluttering
- Delegation of duties

- Changing of looks
- Lessening time on social media
- Etc.

Sample Resolutions

Sample #1: Fitness-related

"I will work out every Monday to Thursday at [name of gym] from 6:00 am to 7:30 am from January 2nd to December 24th and aim to lose at least 70 pounds."

Sample #2: Work-related

"I will delegate Thursday noon meetings to [name of a volunteer] from August to November so I can enjoy vacation with my family for the purposes of family unity and bonding."

Sample #3: Financial-related

"I will save $20 every pay from June to November so I can provide good Christmas gifts to my children to make them happy and feel loved."

Sample #4: Religiously-related

"I will fast (abstain from food), fully abstaining from solid foods every weekend, except on public holiday weekends, from May 1st to July 31st this year to concentrate on understanding the meaning of God's grace."

Sample #5: Academically-related

"I will study Mathematics every Mondays and Wednesdays from 7:00 pm to 10:00 pm from January 21st to May 31st to be ready to ace the subject during the June 14th final examination to get a reasonable GPA for entrance into university science courses."

Sample #6: Politically-related

"I will spend twenty hours per week, ten hours on Mondays and ten more hours on Thursdays, from September 1st to June 30th this year to make calls to my constituent members to hear and respond to their concerns."

Conclusion

Resolutions, and the most popular new year's, are strong decisions made through a promise to adhere to some defined objectives. They must be implemented to achieve a desirable result. There will always be impediments and discouragements on the way, but the resolutioner must be determined, decisive, disciplined and dutiful enough to overcome any challenge to better, improve or actualize themselves through the attainment of the resolution.

ABOUT THE AUTHOR

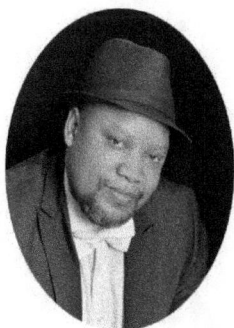

Award-Winning, Best-Selling Author, Charles Mwewa (LLB; BA Law; BA Ed; LLM), is a prolific researcher, poet, novelist, lawyer, law professor and Christian apologist and intercessor. Mwewa has written no less than 100 books and counting in every genre and has exhibited his works at prestigious expos like the Ottawa International Book Expo and is the winner of the Coppa Awards for his signature publication, *Zambia: Struggles of My People.*
Mwewa and his family live in the Canadian Capital City of Ottawa.

SELECTED BOOKS BY THIS AUTHOR

1. *ZAMBIA: Struggles of My People (First and Second Editions)*
2. *10 FINANCIAL & WEALTH ATTITUDES TO AVOID*
3. *10 STRATEGIES TO DEFEAT STRESS AND DEPRESSION: Creating an Internal Safeguard against Stress and Depression*
4. *100+ REASONS TO READ BOOKS*
5. *A CASE FOR AFRICA?S LIBERTY: The Synergistic Transformation of Africa and the West into First-World Partnerships*
6. *DECOLONIZATION: Reclaiming African Originality and Destiny*
7. *A PANDEMIC POETRY, COVID-19*
8. *ALLERGIC TO CORRUPTION: The Legacy of President Michael Sata of Zambia*
9. *BOOK ABOUT SOMETHING: On Ultimate Purpose*
10. *CAMPAIGN FOR AFRICA: A Provocative Crusade for the Economic and Humanitarian Decolonization of Africa*
11. *CHAMPIONS: Application of Common Sense and Biblical Motifs to Succeed in Both*

INDEX

F

falling plane conception, 8
family, 15
Family time and bonding, 11
Finances, 11

G

goals, 4, 10
God, 19

H

habit, 5

I

implementation, 2, 3, 8
individual, 3, 9, 10
internal, 5

L

law, 15
lawyer, 15
looks, 12

M

masks, 8
Mental health, 11

N

negligence, 4
new skills, 11
new things, 11
New year's, 11

O

objectives, vii, 9, 10, 14
oneself, 7
oversight, 4

P

permanence, 10
plans, 1, 2, 3
poet, 15
possibility, 6
professor, 15
project, 4, 5
prolific, 15

Q

question, 7

www.ingramcontent.com/pod-product-compliance
Lightning Source LLC
Chambersburg PA
CBHW060705280326
41933CB00012B/2316